END OF

LIFE IS LIFE

A Hospice Nurse Insight on the

Misconception of the End

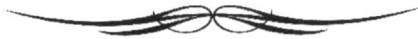

DUNSTEADLER RN, MA

NOTE: This book is intended only as an informative guide for those wishing to know about end of life care. Readers are advised to consult with their doctor/hospice provider. The reader assumes all responsibility for the consequences of any actions taken based on the information presented in this book. The information in this book is based on the author's experience. Every attempt has been made to ensure that the information is accurate; however, the author cannot accept liability for another person's actions.

DEDICATED

This book is dedicated to my Lord Jesus Christ.

Thank you for being my potter.

To my 3%, thank you for your unconditional love

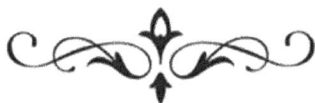

and support.

TABLE OF CONTENTS

CHAPTER 1

INTRODUCTION

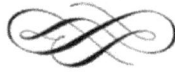

Greetings!

During the summer of 2001, I graduated from Boston College with a Bachelor's Degree. In the fall of that year, I entered graduate school and finished my Master's degree in Organizational/Industrial Psychology. After my Master's Degree, I worked in Human Resources for a few years. Although I enjoyed my job, I desired a career that would bless me with the opportunity to have more influence and impact on individual's lives. I remember going into my closet (my safe haven) and praying to God for guidance. Eventually, the idea of nursing came to mind.

Prior to being accepted into nursing school, I continued working my full-time HR job during the day. After work, I would drive in rush hour traffic to take classes to satisfy my prerequisites in order to be accepted into nursing school. I did this while simultaneously working as an overnight counselor in a group home. This was my schedule for about two years. In 2008, I got accepted into nursing school and left my HR position. I decided to remain in the group home, where I was responsible for passing out medications to the residents and maintaining their safety.

My first nursing job in 2010 was at a rehabilitation hospital. While there, I quickly learned that most nurses have two jobs, and decided to obtain a part-time position at a skilled nursing facility. There, I was fortunate to build relationships with several hospice nurses who would come to the facility to help manage our patients' symptoms and comfort, especially when it comes to pain management. Although I was the primary floor nurse assigned to the patients, I soon realized that the hospice nurses are also known as case managers were more involved, and had more autonomy, connections with the family, and the capability to spend more quality one-on-one time with the patient. Whereas, I often had to manage several patients at the same time and did not quite have the intimate time that I wanted to dedicate individually to each patient. In 2012, I decided to submit and listen to that inner voice inside of me and begin my journey as a Registered Hospice Nurse. Ever since then, I've never looked back. This was one of the best decisions I could have ever made in my life!

The world we live in views dying as fearful and taboo. Something to not ever talk about. Most of us believe that if you say the word "die," it will expedite death. Some family will say "don't use the word hospice." In this book, my goal is to decrease the level of anxiety by just a notch. Realizing that the minute you're born, our end of life clock begins. The moment we are born, we are dying. Just like we would expect a young boy; Dunsson at some point to grow a mustache which is the natural process of life, we too should expect death as a natural process of life.

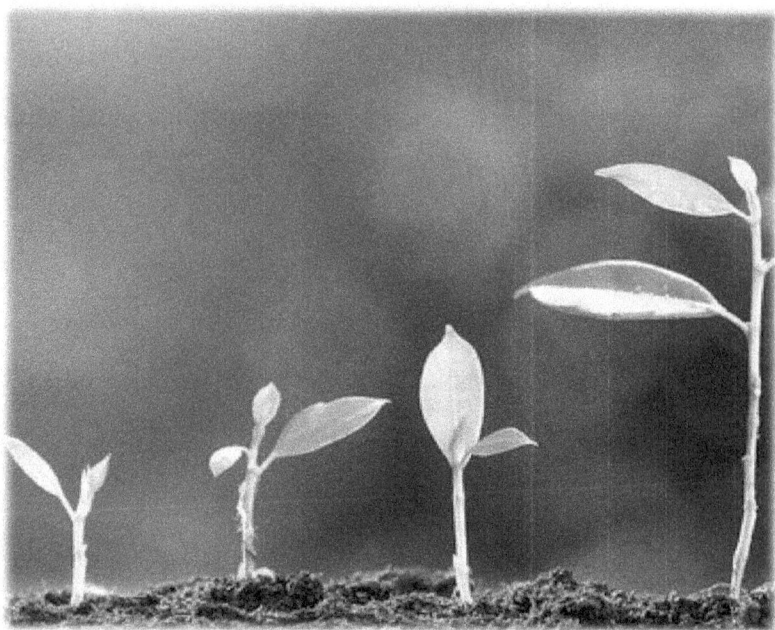

CHAPTER 2

WHAT IS END OF LIFE

HOSPICE CARE

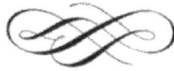

D octors might suggest hospice care after they have exhausted all aggressive treatments. In spite of treatments, the disease is still progressing. The medical experts deem you no longer a candidate for further aggressive treatment. They might say that treatment will cause more harm than good to your body. The moment has come to focus on the **quality** of life versus **quantity.**

Mr Petes

For example, let's introduce 75-year-old, Mr. Petes, with a past medical history of smoking. He has quit smoking now for the past 10 years. About 6 months ago, he began to experience difficulty breathing, increased lethargy, coughing, and unexplained weight loss. Over the past two months, symptoms began to worsen. He finally agreed with his wife, Rosie, to a doctor's visit. Chest X-ray revealed several nodules in both lungs. To confirm, the medical doctor ordered a biopsy, and CT-Scan confirmed metastatic NonSmall Cell Lung Cancer. Immediately, his oncologist started treatment with chemotherapy and radiation. A year later, despite treatment, the masses are growing and the oncologist told Mr. Petes that the aggressive treatments are no longer working and that he's no longer a candidate for aggressive treatment. Mr. Petes no longer wants hospital visits. Last time he was hospitalized, he developed hospital-acquired pneumonia (HAP). Rosie, his wife is starting to feel burnt-out. She worries that she will not be able to safely handle his care by herself at home. She is not sure how to best manage her husband's symptoms. What can the Petes do? The best resource would be hospice care at this time.

Mrs. Doll

Another example, imagine you are taking care of your 82-year-old mother, Mrs. Doll with Alzheimer's dementia. Over the past year, she has been diagnosed with UTIs, pneumonia, and her weight has fluctuated. Now, she is increasingly disoriented, unable to make her needs known, or follow instructions. Total dependent with all personal care. She begins to pocket food in her mouth. Mrs. Doll has lost the ability to walk independently. The other day while changing her diaper, you noticed a reddened area on her coccyx. Mrs. Doll now has lost the ability to ambulate independently. She is having frequent falls and increased episodes of agitation/anxiety. Mrs. Doll had developed three UTIs in the past year. Each time you take her to the hospital, she becomes more anxious and agitated, only to be sent home with little to no solution. Mom is not getting any better; her dementia is progressing and you don't want to keep on taking her back and forth to the hospital. What support is there? The best resource would also be hospice care.

Hospice provides specialized services in managing complex symptoms caused by advanced diseases. Hospice does not mean you're going to die today. This is one of the biggest misconceptions I have heard families assume. From my experience, our patients on average tend to live a longer more comfortable life. As a matter of fact, research has shown that people who are under hospice care live longer and more fulfilled lives. The reason is because of all of the added support that a person receives under hospice care. According to the research journal on American Family Physician, (Am Fam Physician. 2018 Mar 1;97(5):online.) Scientists found that just one day on hospice has the potential to increase one's life by three months.

Hospice is available for added support to help educate, train, and manage end of life symptoms. Hospice nurses are available 24 hours, 7 days a week--even on Christmas Day. Each patient is assigned a primary nurse who will be the main nurse to facilitate your care and manage your symptoms. This nurse will provide weekly visits, coordinate a plan of care that is individually cater to the patient needs. Other important team members include social workers, spiritual coordinators, Hospice aides, Hospice MD, volunteers, and bereavement care. All of these wonderful services aid in providing emotional support to your loved ones. The hospice aide helps with personal care and oftentimes becomes like family. I sometimes hear family members stating, "I will cancel a nursing visit, but please don't take away our Suzette, my hospice aide." Several hospices provide music, massages, and pet therapy. The hospice volunteers who themselves are usually family members who once had a loved one under hospice care, and had such a positive experience with hospice, that they want to support another family member and be a shining light. In addition, the Hospice Medical Director is the physician who will collaborate with your primary care physician to not only facilitate the best-individualized care for you, but is available 24/7 to write scripts of medications that can readily be delivered straight to your front door. For example, if Mr. Petes, who is diagnosed with lung cancer is experiencing difficulty breathing and runs out of his Oxycodone on a Saturday at 1 PM, the hospice medical director is right there to write a new script so that dad does not have to wait until Monday to call his PCP in order to get comfortable. Plus, oxygen can also be delivered that same day. Another blessed support is the readily available medical equipment--such as oxygen concentrators/ portables, hospital beds, wheelchairs, walker air mattresses, diapers, etc. that can be delivered all in one day. You'll often hear me tell my patients, "It's best to have something and not need it than to need something and not have it."

All of the above examples are awesome services that hospice provides. They help to increase a patient's quality of life and alleviates the stress of caregivers. These services can be performed at a patient's home, skilled nursing homes, assisted living facilities, and sometimes directly in the hospital. Best of all, everything is 100% free, covered by your health insurance!

*Hospice care is individualized specialized services in managing end of life symptoms.

* Hospice don't hasten the dying process

*Quality vs. Quantity

CHAPTER 3

WHY HOSPICE NOW RATHER THAN LATER

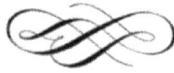

A s shared in the previous chapter, hospice provides several great benefits to both the patient and caregiver. Unfortunately, in most cases, I see that families will wait until the very end when the person is on their deathbed before they call hospice. Sadly, by then the individual is unable to reap all of the benefits explained earlier, and much more that Hospice Care has to offer. The best practice is to contact hospice at the beginning, rather than at the end. For instance, if you or a family member are in a similar situation as Mr. Petes, it would greatly benefit him/her to contact hospice soon after having been told by the MD that there's no treatment available for your diagnosis. The hospice team now has time to plan and design an individualized plan of care in order for Mr. Petes to achieve maximum quality of life.

The best plan of care can be achieved when collaboration exists between the patient, family/caregivers, and the hospice team. The family and the teamwork form an alliance to communicate and interact in such a way that will optimally provide the best care for the patient. As in the case of Mrs. Doll, her pressure ulcer would most likely not worsen if her family willing to place her under hospice care sooner. This is because she would have weekly wound care nursing visits, which can be 2x-5x/week depending on the established plan of care for Mrs. Doll. Her falls might be minimized due to the added safety teaching and equipment that hospice care provides. Another great service might be managing mom's medications. Hospice care can provide medications that will decrease the level of agitation and anxiety that Mrs. Doll is manifesting. Hospice nurses can medicate and also properly teach the family how to facilitate medication for Mrs. Doll, including doses and frequency to keep her comfortable and avoid hospitalization. Moreover, in managing her UTI's, a hospice nurse can obtain a urine sample from mom in the comfort of her home. Afterwards, the hospice nurse will bring the urine sample to a local laboratory. Once the result is obtained, nurse collaborate with the Hospice MD who will fax over a script of the best antibiotics to the hospice affiliate pharmacy, and have it be delivered straight to your door! This is a great service allowing patients to avoid having to make an unnecessary trip to the hospital.

*Allow time to plan and coordinate an individualized plan of care

CHAPTER 4

HOW TO WELCOME OPTIMAL

QUALITY OF LIFE AT END OF LIFE

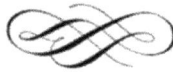

K now that it's perfectly acceptable to be fearful of the unknown. There's no one in the world, presently alive who has been dead, buried, and came back to talk about the experience. I recall at the early stage of my career as a hospice nurse, 94-year-old *Ms. Boyer* stated, "I'm afraid to die." My first thought was...If God ever blesses me with ninety-four years on this Earth, it would be ungrateful of me to ask for more. As the weeks went by, I later discovered that it wasn't dying that she was afraid of, rather, her concerns were not wanting to experience pain. She also expressed her thoughts, fearing that she would suffocate. Moreover, Ms. Boyer had an estranged relationship with her son. Once the hospice team was able to gain her trust and with her permission, I was able to manage her symptoms, pain, and difficulty breathing. Collaborating with the social worker and spiritual coordinator, she was able to have a conversation with her son. In the end, I recall her stating, "I'm ready." Ms. Boyer was able to live her optimal quality of life once her physical and emotional needs were met.

Regarding living the best quality of life under hospice care, we must live in the present. It's a disadvantage to live in either the past or the future of what's to come. Matthew 6:34 reads, *"Therefore do not be anxious about tomorrow, for tomorrow will worry about itself."* Each day has enough trouble of its own. Often, it's not dying that we are afraid of. But, sometimes we have regrets, we feel that we have not accomplished much in life, and/or we are afraid that the world will forget about us/lack of legacy. We might have broken, unresolved relationships with loved ones. We are afraid we will not live to see our children or grandchildren grow up. I encourage all of us to acknowledge these emotions and then release them. Let go of what's out of our control and focus on the present moment. Know that everything happens for a reason, unbeknownst to man.

Hospice care encourages caregivers to spend as much quality time as possible with their loved ones. Optimal quality of life is individualized to meet family needs. For some, it could be the courage to hold dad's hand by his bedside, letting him know just how much you love him, and granting him permission to pass away in peace. Other's could be managing their pain level so that dad is able to be involve when the grandchildren visit. Quality of life for a couple who has been waking up each day for the last 30 years together, and going for a walk might now be the situation where under hospice care now, Mr. Smith drives his wife around while she is utilizing her portable oxygen tank. Although Mrs. Smith with end-stage COPD, lacks the energy to walk around the neighborhood with her husband, she still finds fulfillment in being able to participate in a car ride with her loving husband.

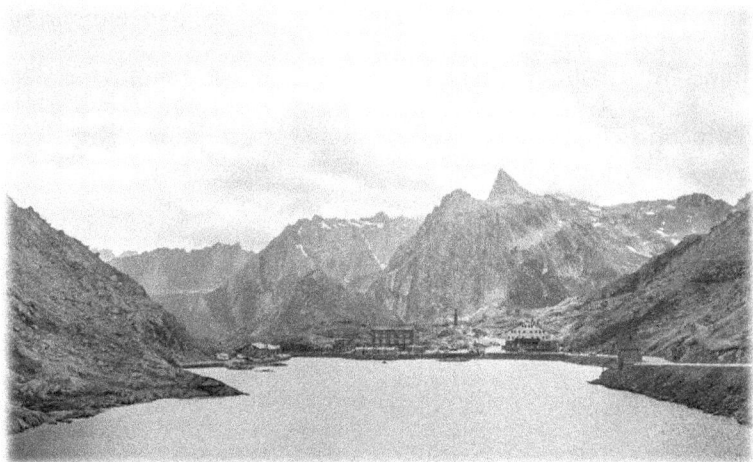

While your loved one may be under hospice care, we still have the choice and can choose to live day-by-day as joyful and fulfilling as possible. Every day is a blessing. That blessing can be as simple as wanting to be pain-free at your children's wedding. You can still travel and be in hospice. Some of the hospice patients have traveled to different states or hours away to attend family functions. For example, if the patient's daughter is getting married and the father's wish is to attend the wedding, this can be coordinated, considering that the patient has the strength and his doctor provides him with clearance to do so. The hospice nurse can coordinate to pack his medications also. Furthermore, if the destination is in a location that is out of the service area of your primary hospice, the hospice team can coordinate with another hospice company and temporarily connect dad with another local hospice company that is near the destination. This way, there will be no interruption in receiving quality care.

Hospice will go above and beyond to make sure that each patient is living their best quality of life. This experience is individualized to cater to each person's needs. The method in which this is best achieved is to focus on one day at a time. Try not to allow the end determine how you live and treat your loved one today. The number one question I get asked as a hospice nurse is, "Dawn, can you tell me when my mom/dad is going to die? Can you tell me how much longer?" I usually reply by saying something to bring light into the situation. I would respond, "Wow if I can predict the answer to that question, I'd tell you tonight's lottery number!" Immediately, I could see the caregiver smile; bringing some light back into the room.

* Live in the present

*Take it one day at a time

CHAPTER 5

CELEBRATING LIFE UNTIL

THE END

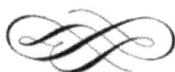

Life is a gift worth celebrating even until the end. I think of it as a marathon runner race. At the beginning of the race, the runner feels strong, energetic, and full of excitement. By the middle of the race, she might begin to feel tired, weak, and have doubts. She may wonder, "Can I make it to the finishing line?" "Am I strong enough?" Then, she reaches the finishing line feeling a great sense of accomplishment and relief. She might not have won first place, but in her mind, she did it. She was able to carry through and not give up, even when there were moments she probably wanted to.

Most of us start this journey we call life with a supernatural mindset...full of energy, believing that we can achieve greatness and do all things. Philippians 4:13 reads, *"I can do everything through Christ who gives me strength."* Then, somewhere in the middle, we embark on some hardships happening in our lives, losses, and disappointments. It might be a divorce, loss of a child, losing your business, getting fired from a job you've worked for years, having an addiction, or losing a pet dog. Whatever the situation is, we wonder, What is the lesson to learn in all of this? Is there a purpose?

As a Hospice nurse having been blessed by hundreds of families over the years who have opened their doors to me and welcomed me into their homes, from sharing some of the deepest sorrows, I learned that the most important thing is Love. Becoming love, and having love in your heart. Being loved by someone. Whether it's the love of a child, spouse, aunt, cousin, a close friend, or your next-door neighbor. At the end of it all, believing that you were created and placed in this world for a purpose. We all can choose to be joyful at the end. We've been provided with the greatest blessing of participating in this marathon race called life. Now, getting to finish it under hospice care. Help us to help you. Go in love, my Love.

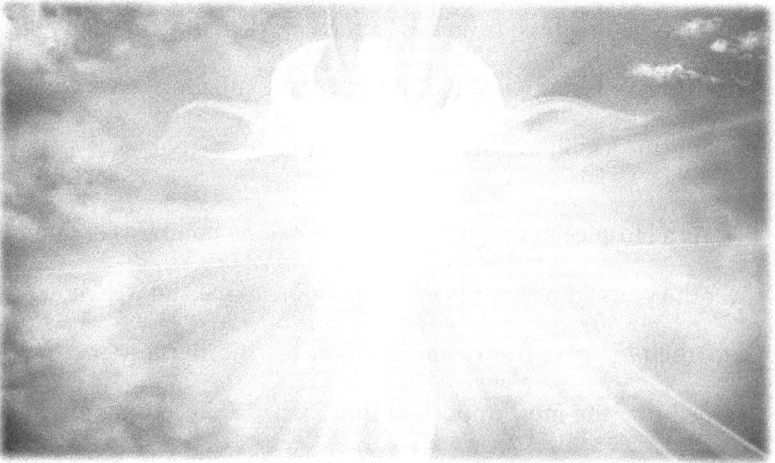

www.ingramcontent.com/pod-product-compliance
Lightning Source LLC
Chambersburg PA
CBHW071126210326
41519CB00020B/6447